THE COMPLETE LOW-FODMAP DIET COOKBOOK FOR BEGINNERS 2024

A Guide to Quick, Easy and Tasty Recipes to Reduce IBS Symptoms and Other Digestive Disorders with 14 Days Meal Plan

TERESA R. THOMAS

Table of Contents

INTRODUCTION

Irritable bowel syndrome (IBS) is a chronic disorder that affects one in every ten individuals worldwide. Symptoms include stomach discomfort and bloating, excessive gas, and frequent diarrhea or constipation. Although physicians can diagnose the issue, they have little success in resolving it.

This book is ideal for anyone suffering from IBS, food intolerances, or other chronic digestive issues who are tired of feeling ill. The low-FODMAP diet has been scientifically demonstrated to alleviate IBS symptoms. This program has successfully improved countless people's lives and has the potential to help you as well.

FODMAP refers to fermentable, poorly absorbed short-chain carbohydrates that feed intestinal bacteria and may induce digestive pain. FODMAP stands for Fermentable Oligosaccharides, Disaccharides, Monosaccharides, and Polyols.

If this terminology is confusing, keep in mind that "saccharide" simply means "sugar." Carbohydrates include Oligosaccharides, Disaccharides, and Monosaccharides. Polyols are sugar alcohols, which are sugar molecules with an alcohol side chain.

This book will go into deeper information about FODMAPs and the low-FODMAP diet. We will guide you through a tailored low-FODMAP diet based on your specific food intolerances and preferences, including which items are safe, which may be consumed in moderation, and which should be avoided entirely.

For now, here are some important things regarding the diet:

- It's been scientifically confirmed.

- It contains all of the essential nutrients.

- Individualized diets may provide long-term symptom relief, with some individuals experiencing no symptoms for months or years.

- While not a cure for IBS, it may help prevent symptoms from recurring.

We believe that adopting the low-FODMAP diet suggested in this book will provide significant relief for IBS sufferers. After starting the diet, you may need to refer to the book sometimes, but it will eventually become second nature. You'll feel better than ever without putting too much effort into the "how."

Using the recipes in this book will help you adjust to the diet more smoothly.

Sincere wishes for good health.

CHAPTER 1: UNDERSTANDING THE LOW FODMAP DIET

What are FODMAPs?

FODMAPs are carbohydrates and sugar alcohols that cause digestive issues such as bloating, stomach discomfort, gas, distention, and diarrhea.

Artificial sweeteners, some vegetables and fruits, lactose-containing dairy products, high fructose corn syrup, beans, wheat, and lentils may all contain them.

Although high-FODMAP meals are generally healthful and useful, some individuals may have unpleasant reactions.

FODMAP-rich foods may trigger symptoms of GI illnesses such as IBS, IBD, GERD, celiac disease, and diverticulitis.

There are five types of FODMAPs: Polyols, Fructans, Fructose, Lactose, and Galactans. Polyols found in fruits and vegetables include sugar alcohols such as xylitol, sorbitol, and Mannitol. Fructans may be found in barley, spelled, rye, and wheat, whereas Galactans are found in legumes such as lentils and beans. Fructose, or simple sugar, may be found in table sugar, fruits, vegetables, and additional sweeteners. Finally, lactose is the primary carbohydrate in dairy products, particularly milk.

What is the Low Fodmap Diet?

The Low FODMAP Diet treats symptoms of irritable bowel syndrome (IBS). IBS, a prevalent gastrointestinal illness, affects around 10-15% of the worldwide population. Symptoms may include bloating, gas, stomach discomfort, constipation, or diarrhea. FODMAPs, a kind of carbohydrate, have been linked to IBS symptoms in certain individuals, while the exact explanation remains unknown.

The abbreviation FODMAP refers to fermentable oligosaccharides, disaccharides, Monosaccharides, and polyols. These carbohydrates are poorly absorbed in the small intestine and quickly fermented by bacteria in the large intestine, causing gas and other symptoms.

The Low FODMAP Diet is a three-phase elimination diet that begins with eliminating high FODMAP foods and gradually reintroduces them to discover triggers. The diet aims to identify and remove trigger foods while maintaining a nutritious balance.

The elimination phase involves removing high FODMAP items from the diet for 4-6 weeks. This includes wheat, onions, garlic, dairy, legumes, and certain fruits including apples, cherries, and peaches. A low FODMAP diet does not exclude gluten, however certain high FODMAP foods, like wheat, may include gluten.

After elimination, FODMAPs are progressively reintroduced, one kind at a time. This identifies trigger foods and FODMAPs that may be tolerated in tiny quantities.

Identifying trigger foods allows for a tailored low FODMAP diet that manages symptoms while remaining nutritionally balanced.

Who Should follow the Low-Fodmap Diet?

This diet is not intended for weight reduction, but rather for persons with IBS or other GI disorders.

Avoid this diet if you do not have a GI problem since it may hurt your health. FODMAPs are prebiotics, which promote healthy gut flora development.

While the low-FODMAP diet may alleviate symptoms, it is not intended to cure autoimmune illnesses. If you're uncertain, talk to your doctor first.

Benefits of The Low-Fodmap Diet

1. The Low-FODMAP Diet may alleviate digestive problems such as bloating, gas, stomach discomfort, constipation, and diarrhea. The diet reduces the consumption of fermentable carbs, which might induce unpleasant symptoms.

2. Improved Nutrient Absorption: The Low-FODMAP Diet reduces digestive discomfort, leading to better nutrient absorption. IBS may induce nutritional malabsorption, potentially leading to malnutrition.

3. Improved Mood: Research indicates that IBS patients are more prone to feel anxiety and despair. The Low-FODMAP Diet may enhance happiness and quality of life by alleviating digestive issues.

4. Increased Dietary Variety: The Low-FODMAP diet restricts specific foods but promotes intake of a diverse range of low-FODMAP foods. This may result in a more diversified and balanced diet.

5. Improved Quality of Life: The Low-FODMAP Diet may enhance the quality of life for IBS patients by lowering digestive symptoms and increasing overall health. This may improve productivity, social involvement, and well-being.

Recommended Foods for a Low-Fodmap Diet

1. All oil and fats.

2. Vegetables: yams, water chestnuts, kale, radishes, spinach, celery, turnips, bamboo shoots, lettuce, alfalfa sprouts, potatoes, zucchini, ginger, squash, sweet potatoes, bean sprouts, parsnips, eggplant, chives, bell peppers, cucumbers, bok choy, carrots, olives, green beans, and tomatoes.

3. Low FODMAP fruits include mandarins, passion fruit, raspberries, strawberries, cantaloupes, grapes, lime, oranges, grapefruit, honeydew melons, oranges, bananas, kiwi, blueberries, and lemons.

4. Lactose-free dairy options include aged soft cheeses (such as camembert and brie) and hard cheeses.

5. Most spices and herbs.

6. Proteins with low FODMAP content include beef, pig, poultry, fish, and eggs.

7. Soy, which includes tofu and tempeh.

8. Grains you may consume include maize, oats, rice, quinoa, sorghum, and tapioca.

9. Gluten-free foods include bread, pasta, rice, oat bran, quinoa, sourdough, rice bran, and cornflour. Gluten is not a FODMAP, however many gluten-free items are low in FODMAPs.

10. This group includes beverages including almond milk, rice milk, tea, coffee, non-concentrated fruit juice, and water.

11. Protein-rich nuts and seeds include almonds, macadamia, peanuts, pine nuts, walnuts, sesame seeds, and pumpkin seeds. Consume simply a few of them every day for optimal results. Overeating leads to increased absorption of FODMAPs.

Foods to Eat

1. **Low-FODMAP fruits:** Opt for fruits such as berries (strawberries, blueberries, raspberries), citrus fruits (oranges, lemons, limes), grapes, kiwi, and pineapple. These fruits are lower in FODMAPs and less likely to trigger symptoms.

2. **Vegetables:** Stick to non-cruciferous vegetables like spinach, zucchini, carrots, cucumber, bell peppers, tomatoes, and potatoes. These vegetables are generally well-tolerated and provide essential vitamins and minerals.

3. **Protein sources:** Choose lean proteins like chicken, turkey, fish, tofu, tempeh, and eggs. These proteins are low in FODMAPs and can help meet your daily protein needs.

4. **Grains:** Opt for gluten-free grains such as rice (white, brown, or wild), quinoa, oats (certified gluten-free), and corn. These grains are safe for a low-FODMAP diet and provide fiber and energy.

5. **Dairy Alternatives:** If lactose intolerant, choose lactose-free or dairy-free alternatives like lactose-free milk, almond milk, coconut milk, and lactose-free yogurt. These options provide calcium and other nutrients without triggering symptoms.

6. **Nuts and Seeds:** Stick to low-FODMAP nuts and seeds such as almonds, walnuts, peanuts (in moderation), pumpkin seeds, and sunflower seeds. These can be consumed in small portions as snacks or added to meals for extra nutrients and texture.

7. **Fats and oils:** Use olive oil, coconut oil, and other low-FODMAP oils for cooking and dressing salads. These healthy fats provide energy and aid in a variety of biological activities.

Foods to Avoid

1. **High-FODMAP fruits:** Avoid fruits such as apples, pears, mangoes, cherries, watermelons, and stone fruits like peaches and plums. These fruits

are high in FODMAPs and can exacerbate symptoms.

2. **Certain vegetables:** Limit intake of high-FODMAP vegetables like onions, garlic, cauliflower, broccoli, asparagus, and Brussels sprouts. These vegetables contain fermentable carbohydrates that can cause digestive distress.

3. **Legumes:** Avoid legumes such as beans, lentils, chickpeas, and soybeans, as they are high in FODMAPs and can contribute to gas and bloating.

4. **Dairy Products:** Steer clear of high-lactose dairy products like milk, soft cheeses, yogurt, and ice cream. These dairy products can worsen symptoms in individuals with lactose intolerance.

5. **Wheat and Rye Products:** Eliminate foods containing wheat and rye, including bread, pasta, cereals, and baked goods. These grains contain high levels of fructans, a type of FODMAP that can trigger symptoms.

6. **Sweeteners:** Avoid artificial sweeteners like sorbitol, mannitol, xylitol, and maltitol, which are high in polyols and can cause gastrointestinal discomfort.

7. **Processed Foods:** Read labels carefully and avoid processed foods that contain high-FODMAP ingredients like honey, high-fructose corn syrup, inulin, and certain additives and preservatives.

By focusing on low-FODMAP foods and avoiding high-FODMAP triggers, individuals can effectively manage their symptoms while still achieving a balanced and nutritious diet. It's essential to work with a healthcare professional or registered dietitian to ensure nutritional adequacy and long-term dietary sustainability.

CHAPTER 2

Breakfast Recipes

1. Coconut Cacao Hazelnut Smoothie Bowl

Ingredients:

- 1 ripe banana, frozen

- 1/4 cup coconut milk

- 2 tablespoons cacao powder

- 1 tablespoon hazelnut butter

- 1/4 cup rolled oats

- Toppings: sliced banana, cacao nibs, shredded coconut, chopped hazelnuts

Preparation:

1. In a blender, combine the frozen banana, coconut milk, cacao powder, hazelnut butter, and rolled oats. Blend until smooth.

2. Transfer the smoothie to a bowl.

3. Top with sliced banana, cacao nibs, shredded coconut, and chopped hazelnuts.

Nutritional Value (per serving):

- Calories: 380

- Protein: 7g

- Fat: 20g

- Carbohydrates: 47g

- Fiber: 8g

- Sugar: 17g

Cooking Time: 5 minutes

Number of Servings: 1

2. Summer Berry Smoothie

Ingredients:

- One cup mixed berries (strawberries, raspberries, blueberries).

- 1/2 cup Greek yogurt

- 1/2 cup almond milk

- 1 tablespoon honey or maple syrup

- 1/2 teaspoon vanilla extract

Preparation:

1. In a blender, combine the mixed berries, Greek yogurt, almond milk, honey or maple syrup, and vanilla extract. Blend until smooth.

2. Pour into glasses and serve immediately.

Nutritional Value (per serving):

- Calories: 150

- Protein: 8g

- Fat: 2g

- Carbohydrates: 28g

- Fiber: 6g

- Sugar: 20g

Cooking Time: 5 minutes

Number of Servings: 2

3. Basic Smoothie Base

Ingredients:

- 1 ripe banana

- 1/2 cup frozen mixed berries

- 1/2 cup spinach leaves

- 1/2 cup almond milk

- 1/4 cup Greek yogurt

- 1 tablespoon chia seeds (optional)

Preparation:

1. In a blender, combine the banana, frozen mixed berries, spinach leaves, almond milk, Greek yogurt, and chia seeds (if using). Blend until smooth.

2. Add more almond milk if needed to reach desired consistency.

Nutritional Value (per serving):

- Calories: 180

- Protein: 6g

- Fat: 5g

- Carbohydrates: 30g

- Fiber: 8g

- Sugar: 16g

Cooking Time: 5 minutes

Number of Servings: 2

4. Cheese And Herb Scones

Ingredients:

- 2 cups all-purpose flour

- 2 teaspoons baking powder

- 1/2 teaspoon salt.

- 1/4 cup cold, diced unsalted butter.

- 1 cup grated cheddar cheese

- 2 tablespoons chopped fresh herbs (parsley, chives, or thyme)

- 3/4 cup milk

- One beaten egg for the egg wash.

Preparation:

1. Preheat the oven to 400°F (200°C). Line a baking sheet with parchment paper.

2. In a large basin, combine the flour, baking powder, and salt.

3. Cut in the cold butter using a pastry cutter or fork until the mixture resembles coarse crumbs.

4. Stir in the grated cheese and chopped herbs.

5. Gradually add the milk, stirring until the dough comes together.

6. Turn the dough out onto a lightly floured surface and knead gently a few times until smooth.

7. Shape the dough into a 1-inch-thick round. Cut into wedges and arrange on the prepared baking sheet.

8. Brush the beaten egg on the tops of the scones.

9. Bake for 15–18 minutes, or until golden brown.

Nutritional Value (per serving - 1 scone):

- Calories: 220

- Protein: 7g

- Fat: 11g

- Carbohydrates: 24g

- Fiber: 1g

- Sugar: 1g

Cooking Time: 20 minutes

Number of Servings: 8 scones

5. Brownie Pancakes

Ingredients:

- 1 cup all-purpose flour

- 1/4 cup unsweetened cocoa powder

- 1/4 cup granulated sugar

- 1 teaspoon baking powder

- 1/2 teaspoon baking soda

- 1/4 teaspoon salt

- 1 cup buttermilk

- 1 large egg

- 2 tablespoons melted butter

- 1 teaspoon vanilla extract

- Chocolate chips (optional, for topping)

Preparation:

1. In a large bowl, whisk together the flour, cocoa powder, sugar, baking powder, baking soda, and salt.

2. In another bowl, whisk together the buttermilk, egg, melted butter, and vanilla extract.

3. Add the wet ingredients to the dry ones and whisk until just blended.

4. Place a nonstick skillet or griddle over medium heat. Apply a little layer of butter or cooking spray.

5. Pour about 1/4 cup batter into the griddle for each pancake.

6. Cook until bubbles form on the surface, then flip and cook until the other side is cooked through.

7. Serve warm, topped with chocolate chips if desired.

Nutritional Value (per serving - 2 pancakes):

- Calories: 300

- Protein: 8g

- Fat: 10g

- Carbohydrates: 46g

- Fiber: 3g

- Sugar: 16g

Cooking Time: 15 minutes

Number of Servings: 4 servings (8 pancakes)

6. Carrot and Walnut Salad

Ingredients:

- 4 cups grated carrots

- 1/2 cup chopped walnuts

- 1/4 cup raisins

- 2 tablespoons lemon juice

- 2 tablespoons olive oil

- 1 tablespoon honey

- Salt and pepper to taste

- Garnish with fresh parsley or cilantro (optional).

Preparation:

1. In a large bowl, combine the grated carrots, chopped walnuts, and raisins.

2. In a small mixing bowl, combine the lemon juice, olive oil, honey, salt, and pepper.

3. Pour the dressing over the carrot mixture and toss to coat.

4. Garnish with fresh parsley or cilantro if desired.

Nutritional Value (per serving):

- Calories: 200

- Protein: 4g

- Fat: 14g

- Carbohydrates: 20g

- Fiber: 5g

- Sugar: 12g

Preparation Time: 10 minutes

Number of Servings: 4 servings

7. Thai Pumpkin Noodle Soup

Ingredients:

- 1 tablespoon coconut oil

- 1 small onion, chopped

- 2 cloves garlic, minced

- 1 tablespoon grated ginger

- 2 cups pumpkin puree

- 4 cups vegetable broth

- One can (14 ounces) coconut milk

- Two teaspoons of Thai red curry paste.

- 2 tablespoons soy sauce

- 2 tablespoons lime juice

- 8 oz rice noodles

- Salt and pepper to taste

- Fresh cilantro for garnish.

Preparation:

1. In a large saucepan, melt the coconut oil over medium heat. Add the chopped onion and simmer until it softens.

2. Stir in the minced garlic and grated ginger, cooking for another minute until fragrant.

3. Stir in the pumpkin puree, vegetable broth, coconut milk, Thai red curry paste, soy sauce, and lime juice. Bring to a simmer.

4. Cook the rice noodles according to the package directions until soft.

5. Add salt and pepper to taste.

6. Serve hot and garnish with fresh cilantro.

Nutritional Value (per serving):

- Calories: 350

- Protein: 6g

- Fat: 15g

- Carbohydrates: 48g

- Fiber: 6g

- Sugar: 5g

Cooking Time: 30 minutes

Number of Servings: 4 servings

CHAPTER 3

Fish and Seafood Recipes

1. Light Tuna Casserole

Ingredients:

- 8 oz (225g) whole wheat pasta

- One can (10.5 oz / 298g) cream of mushroom soup.

- 1 cup (240ml) low-fat milk

- 1 can (6 oz / 170g) chunk light tuna, drained

- 1 cup (150g) frozen peas.

- 1 cup (100g) of shredded cheddar cheese.

- Salt and pepper to taste

Preparation

1. Preheat the oven to 350°F/175°C.

2. Cook the pasta per package directions until al dente, then drain and leave aside.

3. In a large bowl, mix the cream of mushroom soup and milk until well combined.

4. Add the cooked pasta, tuna, frozen peas, and half of the shredded cheddar cheese to the bowl, and stir until everything is evenly coated.

5. Transfer the mixture to a prepared baking dish and top with the remaining cheese.

6. Bake for 25-30 minutes, or until the cheese is bubbly and golden brown.

7. Serve hot and enjoy!

Nutritional value per serving (assuming four servings)

- Calories: Approximately 400

- Protein: Approximately 25g

- Carbohydrates: Approximately 40g

- Fat: Approximately 15g

Cooking Time: Approximately 45 minutes

Number of Servings: 4

2. Rita's Linguine with Clam Sauce

Ingredients:

- 8 oz (225g) linguine

- 2 tbsp olive oil

- 3 cloves garlic, minced

- 1/4 cup (60ml) white wine

- 2 cans (6.5 oz / 184g each) of chopped clams, undrained

- 1/4 cup (10g) freshly chopped parsley.

- Salt and pepper to taste

Preparation:

1. Cook the linguine according to package instructions until al dente, then drain and set aside.

2. Warm the olive oil in a large pan over medium heat. Sauté the minced garlic for about 1-2 minutes, or until aromatic.

3. Pour in the white wine and let it simmer for 2-3 minutes, allowing the alcohol to cook off.

4. Add the chopped clams (with their juices) to the skillet and simmer for another 3-4 minutes.

5. Add the chopped parsley and season with salt and pepper to taste.

6. Add the cooked linguine to the skillet and toss until well combined and heated through.

7. Serve hot, optionally garnished with additional parsley, and enjoy!

Nutritional value per serving (assuming four portions)

- Calories: Approximately 350

- Protein: Approximately 15g

- Carbohydrates: Approximately 40g

- Fat: Approximately 12g

Cooking Time: Approximately 20 minutes

Number of Servings: 4

3. Shrimp Puttanesca With Linguine

Ingredients:

- 8 oz (225g) linguine

- 2 tbsp olive oil

- 3 cloves garlic, minced

- 1/4 cup (50g) chopped red onion

- 1 can (14.5 oz / 411g) diced tomatoes, undrained

- 1/4 cup (50g) sliced Kalamata olives

- 2 tbsp capers

- Half of a teaspoon of red pepper flakes (to taste).

- 1/2 lb (225g) medium shrimp, peeled and deveined

- Salt and pepper to taste

- Chopped fresh parsley for garnish

Preparation:

1. Cook the linguine according to package instructions until al dente, then drain and set aside.

2. Heat the olive oil in a big pan over medium heat. Add the minced garlic and chopped red onion, and sauté until softened about 2-3 minutes.

3. Stir in the diced tomatoes, sliced Kalamata olives, capers, and red pepper flakes. Simmer for 5-7 minutes to enable the flavors to mingle.

4. Add the shrimp to the skillet and cook until pink and opaque, about 3-4 minutes.

5. Add salt and pepper to taste.

6. Add the cooked linguine to the skillet and toss until well coated with the sauce.

7. Serve hot, garnished with chopped fresh parsley.

Nutritional value per serving (assuming four portions).

- Calories: Approximately 350

- Protein: Approximately 20g

- Carbohydrates: Approximately 45g

- Fat: Approximately 10g

Cooking Time: Approximately 25 minutes

Number of Servings: 4

4. Atlantic Cod with Basil

Ingredients:

- 4 Atlantic cod fillets (about 6 oz / 170g each)

- 2 tbsp olive oil

- 2 cloves garlic, minced

- 1/4 cup (10g) chopped fresh basil

- Salt and pepper to taste

- Lemon wedges for serving

Preparation:

1. Preheat your oven to 400°F (200°C).

2. Arrange the fish fillets on a baking pan lined with parchment paper.

3. In a small bowl, mix the olive oil, minced garlic, and chopped fresh basil.

4. Brush the olive oil mixture over the top of each cod fillet.

5. Season the fillets with salt and pepper to taste.

6. Bake in the preheated oven for 12-15 minutes, or until the fish is opaque and flakes easily with a fork.

7. Serve hot, with lemon slices on the side.

Nutritional value per serving (assuming four servings):

- Calories: Approximately 200

- Protein: Approximately 25g

- Carbohydrates: Approximately 1g

- Fat: Approximately 10g

Cooking Time: Approximately 15 minutes

Number of Servings: 4

5. Walnut Sauce

Ingredients:

- 1 cup walnuts

- 2 cloves garlic

- 1/4 cup grated Parmesan cheese

- 1/4 cup olive oil

- Salt and pepper to taste

- 1/2 cup fresh parsley leaves

- 1/2 cup vegetable broth or water

Preparation:

1. Prepare the Walnuts: Toast the walnuts in a dry skillet over medium heat for about 5 minutes, or until fragrant. Be careful not to burn them.

2. Blend Ingredients: In a food processor, combine the toasted walnuts, garlic, Parmesan cheese, olive

oil, salt, pepper, and parsley leaves. Blend until smooth.

3. Adjust Consistency: While blending, gradually add the vegetable broth or water until the sauce reaches your desired consistency.

4. Serve: Use immediately as a sauce for pasta, vegetables, or meat dishes.

Nutritional Value:

- Calories: Approximately 200 calories per serving (1/4 cup)

- Protein: 4 grams

- Fat: 18 grams

- Carbohydrates: 5 grams

- Fiber: 2 grams

Cooking Time and Servings:

Cooking Time: 10 minutes

Servings: Makes about 1 cup of sauce, serving 4 people

6. Coconut Shrimp

Ingredients:

- 1 pound large shrimp, peeled and deveined

- 1 cup shredded coconut

- 1/2 cup bread crumbs

- 2 eggs, beaten

- Salt and pepper to taste

- Cooking oil for frying

Preparation:

1. Prepare Shrimp: Pat the shrimp dry with paper towels and season with salt and pepper.

2. Coat Shrimp: In one bowl, combine the shredded coconut and bread crumbs. In another bowl, beat the eggs. Dip each shrimp in the beaten eggs, then coat it with the coconut mixture.

3. Fry Shrimp: Heat cooking oil in a large skillet over medium-high heat. Fry the coated shrimp in

batches for 2-3 minutes on each side, or until golden brown and crispy.

4. Drain: Remove the shrimp from the skillet and place them on a plate lined with paper towels to drain excess oil.

Nutritional Value:

- Calories: Approximately 250 calories per serving (4 shrimp)

- Protein: 15 grams

- Fat: 15 grams

- Carbohydrates: 15 grams

- Fiber: 2 grams

Cooking Time and Servings:

Cooking Time: 15 minutes

Servings: Makes about 4 servings

7. Shrimp with Cherry Tomatoes

Ingredients:

- 1 pound shrimp, peeled and deveined

- 2 cups cherry tomatoes, halved

- 3 cloves garlic, minced

- 2 tablespoons olive oil

- Salt and pepper to taste

- 1/4 cup fresh basil leaves, chopped

- Lemon wedges for serving

Preparation:

1. Saute Garlic and Tomatoes: Heat olive oil in a large skillet over medium heat. Add the minced garlic and cook for 1 minute, or until fragrant. Add the cherry tomatoes and cook for another 3-4 minutes, until they start to soften.

2. Cook Shrimp: Add the shrimp to the skillet with the tomatoes and garlic. Season with salt and

pepper. Cook for 4-5 minutes, stirring occasionally, until the shrimp are pink and cooked through.

3. Finish: Stir in the chopped basil leaves and cook for an additional minute. Remove from heat.

4. Serve: Serve the shrimp and cherry tomatoes immediately, garnished with lemon wedges.

Nutritional Value:

- Calories: Approximately 180 calories per serving (4 ounces shrimp with tomatoes)

- Protein: 20 grams

- Fat: 8 grams

- Carbohydrates: 6 grams

- Fiber: 2 grams

Cooking Time and Servings:

Cooking Time: 15 minutes

Servings: Makes about 4 servings

CHAPTER 4

Vegetarian and Vegan Recipes

1. Vegan Pad Thai

Ingredients:

- 200g flat rice noodles.

- 200g firm tofu, squeezed and diced.

- 2 tablespoons vegetable oil

- 3 cloves garlic, minced

- 1 small onion, sliced

- 1 red bell pepper, julienned

- 1 carrot, julienned

- 2 cups bean sprouts

- 3 tablespoons soy sauce

- 2 tablespoons maple syrup

- 2 tablespoons lime juice

- To garnish, combine crushed peanuts and chopped cilantro.

Preparation:

1. Cook the rice noodles according to the package directions. Drain and put aside.

2. Warm the vegetable oil in a large pan over medium heat. Cook until both sides of the tofu cubes are golden brown. Remove from skillet and set aside.

3. In the same skillet, add the garlic and onion. Cook until softened, then add the bell pepper and carrot. Cook until the vegetables are tender.

4. Add the cooked noodles, tofu, bean sprouts, soy sauce, maple syrup, and lime juice to the skillet. Toss everything together until fully mixed and cooked through. 5. Serve hot, garnished with crushed peanuts and chopped cilantro.

Nutritional Value:

Serving Size: 1 plate

- Calories: 350

- Protein: 12g

- Carbohydrates: 50g

- Fat: 12g

- Fiber: 5g

Cooking Time: 30 minutes

Number of Servings: 4

2. Orange Tempeh and Rice Salad:

Ingredients:

- 1 cup brown rice, cooked

- 250g tempeh, cubed

- 2 oranges, segmented

- 1 cucumber, diced

- 1 red onion, thinly sliced

- 1/4 cup fresh cilantro, chopped

- 2 tablespoons soy sauce

- 2 tablespoons orange juice

- 1 tablespoon olive oil

- Salt and pepper to taste

Preparation:

1. In a large bowl, combine the cooked brown rice, orange segments, cucumber, red onion, and cilantro.

2. In a separate bowl, whisk together the soy sauce, orange juice, olive oil, salt, and pepper to make the dressing.

3. Heat a skillet over medium heat and add the tempeh cubes. Cook till golden brown on all sides.

4. Add the cooked tempeh to the salad bowl and toss with the dressing until well-coated.

5. Serve chilled or at room temperature.

Nutritional Value:

- Serving Size: 1 bowl

- Calories: 300

- Protein: 15g

- Carbohydrates: 40g

- Fat: 10g

- Fiber: 6g

Cooking Time: 40 minutes

Number of Servings: 3

3. Collard Green Wraps With Thai Peanut Dressing

Ingredients:

- 6 large collard green leaves

- 1 cup cooked quinoa

- 1 red bell pepper, julienned

- 1 carrot, julienned

- 1/2 cucumber, julienned

- 1/4 cup chopped fresh cilantro

- 1/4 cup chopped roasted peanuts

- For the Thai Peanut Dressing:

- 1/4 cup peanut butter

- 2 tablespoons soy sauce

- 1 tablespoon maple syrup

- 1 tablespoon rice vinegar

- 1 teaspoon sesame oil

- 1 clove garlic, minced

- 1 teaspoon grated ginger

- Water to thin, as needed

Preparation:

1. Wash and dry the collard green leaves, then remove the thick stems from each leaf.

2. In a large bowl, mix the cooked quinoa, bell pepper, carrot, cucumber, cilantro, and chopped peanuts.

3. In a separate bowl, whisk together all the ingredients for the Thai Peanut Dressing until

smooth. Add more water as required to get the desired consistency.

4. Lay a collard green leaf flat on a cutting board. Spoon some of the quinoa mixture onto the center of the leaf, then drizzle with the Thai Peanut Dressing.

5. Fold the sides of the collard green leaf over the filling, then roll it up tightly like a burrito. Repeat with what's left of the leaves and filling.

6. Serve immediately, or refrigerate for later.

Nutritional Value:

- Serving Size: 1 wrap

- Calories: 180

- Protein: 8g

- Carbohydrates: 20g

- Fat: 9g

- Fiber: 5g

Cooking Time: 20 minutes

Number of Servings: 6

4. Baked Tofu Bánh Mì Lettuce Wrap

Ingredients:

- 200g extra-firm tofu, sliced into thin strips

- 1 tablespoon soy sauce

- 1 tablespoon rice vinegar

- 1 tablespoon maple syrup

- 1 teaspoon sesame oil

- 1 clove garlic, minced

- 4 large lettuce leaves

- 1/2 cucumber, thinly sliced

- 1/2 carrot, julienned

- 1/4 cup fresh cilantro leaves

- 2 tablespoons vegan mayonnaise

- 2 tablespoons sriracha sauce

Preparation:

1. Preheat your oven to 375°F (190°C).

2. In a small bowl, whisk together the soy sauce, rice vinegar, maple syrup, sesame oil, and minced garlic. Put the tofu strips in a shallow dish and pour the marinade over them. Allow to marinade for at least 15 minutes.

3. Place the marinated tofu strips on a baking sheet lined with parchment paper. Bake in the preheated oven for 20-25 minutes, flipping halfway through, until tofu is golden and crispy.

4. To make the wraps, lay a lettuce leaf on a dish. Top with baked tofu strips, cucumber slices, julienned carrot, and cilantro leaves.

5. In a small bowl, mix the vegan mayonnaise and sriracha sauce. Drizzle over the filling.

6. Serve immediately.

Nutritional Value:

- Serving Size: 1 wrap

- Calories: 150

- Protein: 8g

- Carbohydrates: 10g

- Fat: 8g

- Fiber: 3g

Cooking Time: 40 minutes

Number of Servings: 4

5 - Walnut Sauce

Ingredients:

- 1 cup walnuts

- 2 cloves garlic

- 1/4 cup grated Parmesan cheese

- 1/4 cup olive oil

- Salt and pepper to taste

Nutritional Value (per serving, assuming 4 servings):

- Calories: 250

- Total Fat: 24g

- Saturated Fat: 3g

- Cholesterol: 5mg

- Sodium: 100mg

- Total Carbohydrates: 5g

- Dietary Fiber: 2g

- Sugars: 1g

- Protein: 5g

Preparation:

1. Toast walnuts in a dry skillet over medium heat until fragrant, about 5 minutes.

2. In a food processor, combine toasted walnuts, garlic, and Parmesan cheese. Pulse until finely chopped.

3. With the food processor running, slowly drizzle in the olive oil until the mixture forms a smooth sauce.

4. Add salt and pepper to taste. If necessary, add more olive oil to get the desired consistency. Serve over pasta, roasted vegetables, or grilled chicken.

Cooking Time: 10 minutes

Number of Servings: 4

6. Coconut Shrimp

Ingredients:

- 1 lb big shrimp, scraped and defined.

- 1 cup shredded coconut

- 1 cup panko breadcrumbs

- 2 eggs, beaten

- Salt and pepper to taste

- Oil for frying

Nutritional Value (per serving, assuming 4 servings):

- Calories: 400

- Total Fat: 20g

- Saturated Fat: 15g

- Cholesterol: 200mg

- Sodium: 600mg

- Total Carbohydrates: 25g

- Dietary Fiber: 2g

- Sugars: 2g

- Protein: 30g

Preparation:

1. Toss shrimp with pepper and salt.

2. In separate bowls, place beaten eggs, shredded coconut, and panko breadcrumbs.

3. Dip each shrimp into the beaten eggs, then coat with shredded coconut and finally with panko breadcrumbs.

4. Heat oil in a deep skillet or fryer to 350°F (180°C).

5. Fry shrimp in batches until golden brown and crispy, about 2-3 minutes per side.

6. Eliminate the shrimp from the oil and drain on paper towels. Serve with your favorite dipping sauce.

Cooking Time: 15 minutes

Number of Servings: 4

7. Shrimp with Cherry Tomatoes

Ingredients:

- 1 lb shrimp, peeled and deveined

- 2 cups cherry tomatoes, halved

- 3 cloves garlic, minced

- 2 tablespoons olive oil

- 1/4 cup chopped fresh basil

- Salt and pepper to taste

Nutritional Value (per serving, assuming 4 servings):

- Calories: 200

- Total Fat: 8g

- Saturated Fat: 1g

- Cholesterol: 150mg

- Sodium: 300mg

- Total Carbohydrates: 6g

- Dietary Fiber: 2g

- Sugars: 3g

- Protein: 25g

Preparation:

1. Heat the olive oil in a large pan over medium heat. Cook for approximately 1 minute, or until the garlic is aromatic.

2. Cook the shrimp in the skillet until pink and opaque, approximately 2-3 minutes on each side.

3. Stir in cherry tomatoes and cook until they begin to soften about 2 minutes.

4. Season with salt and pepper to taste, then sprinkle with chopped fresh basil.

5. Serve hot cooked pasta or with crusty bread. Enjoy!

Cooking Time: 10 minutes

Number of Servings: 4

CHAPTER 5

Soups, Salads and Sides

1. Peppered Beef and Citrus Salad

Ingredients:

- 1 lb beef sirloin, thinly sliced

- 2 tablespoons black peppercorns, crushed

- Salt to taste

- 6 cups mixed salad greens

- 2 oranges, peeled and segmented

- 1 grapefruit, peeled and segmented

- 1/4 cup sliced red onion

- 1/4 cup sliced almonds, toasted

- 1/4 cup crumbled feta cheese

- 1/4 cup balsamic vinaigrette

Preparation:

1. Season the beef slices with crushed black peppercorns and salt.

2. Heat a skillet over medium-high heat and cook the beef slices for 2-3 minutes on each side, or until cooked to your desired level of doneness. Take it off the stove and give it some time to rest.

3. In a large bowl, toss together the mixed salad greens, orange segments, grapefruit segments, sliced red onion, toasted almonds, and crumbled feta cheese.

4. Slice the cooked beef thinly and add it to the salad.

5. Pour the salad with the balsamic vinaigrette and toss to mix.

6. Serve immediately.

Nutritional Value: *This salad is rich in protein from the beef, vitamin C from the citrus fruits and healthy fats from the almonds and feta cheese.*

Cooking Time: Approximately 15 minutes

Servings: 4

2. Orange, Red, and Green Buckwheat Salad

Ingredients:

- 1 cup buckwheat groats

- 2 cups water

- 1 orange, peeled and segmented

- 1 red bell pepper, diced

- 1 cucumber, diced

- 1/4 cup chopped fresh parsley

- 1/4 cup crumbled feta cheese

- 2 tablespoons olive oil

- 1 tablespoon lemon juice

- Salt and pepper to taste

Preparation:

1. Rinse the buckwheat groats under cold water and drain.

2. Place two cups of water in a pot and bring to a boil. Add the buckwheat groats, reduce heat to low,

cover, and simmer for 10-12 minutes, or until the buckwheat is tender and water is absorbed. Turn off the heat and let it cool.

3. In a large bowl, combine the cooked buckwheat, orange segments, diced red bell pepper, diced cucumber, chopped parsley, and crumbled feta cheese.

4. Combine the lemon juice, olive oil, salt, and pepper in a small bowl.

5. Drizzle the salad with the dressing and toss to mix.

6. Serve chilled or at room temperature.

Nutritional Value: This salad is a good source of fiber, vitamins, and minerals, including vitamin C from the oranges and bell pepper, and magnesium from the buckwheat.

Cooking Time: Approximately 15 minutes

Servings: 4

3. Baked Papaya and Chicken Salad with Cilantro-Lime Dressing

Ingredients:

- 2 chicken breasts, boneless and skinless

- 2 tablespoons olive oil

- Salt and pepper to taste

- 1 papaya, peeled, seeded, and diced

- 1 avocado, diced

- 1/4 cup chopped fresh cilantro

- Juice of 2 limes

- 2 tablespoons honey

- 1 tablespoon Dijon mustard

- 1 garlic clove, minced

- 1/4 cup olive oil

- Salt and pepper to taste

- Mixed salad greens for serving

Preparation:

1. Preheat the oven to 375°F (190°C).

2. Rub the chicken breasts with olive oil and season with salt and pepper. Put them in the oven for 20 to 25 minutes, or until they are cooked through, on a baking sheet. Let them cool slightly, then slice them thinly.

3. In a large bowl, combine the diced papaya, diced avocado, and chopped cilantro.

4. In a separate small bowl, whisk together the lime juice, honey, Dijon mustard, minced garlic, olive oil, salt, and pepper to make the dressing.

5. Add the sliced chicken to the bowl with the papaya and avocado. Pour the cilantro-lime dressing over the salad and toss to coat.

6. Serve the salad over a bed of mixed salad greens.

***Nutritional Value:** This salad is a good source of lean protein from the chicken, healthy fats from the avocado, and vitamin C from the papaya. The cilantro-lime dressing adds flavor without adding too much fat or calories.*

Cooking Time: Approximately 30 minutes

Servings: 4

4. Chicken Noodle Soup with Bok Choy

Ingredients:

- 8 cups chicken broth

- 2 boneless, skinless chicken breasts

- 2 carrots, sliced

- 2 stalks celery, sliced

- 4 oz dried noodles (such as egg noodles or rice noodles)

- 2 baby bok choy, chopped

- Salt and pepper to taste

- Fresh parsley for garnish

Preparation:

1. Bring the chicken stock to a boil in a large pot.

2. Add the chicken breasts, carrots, and celery to the pot. Reduce heat to medium-low and simmer for 20-25 minutes, or until the chicken is cooked through.

3. Remove the chicken breasts from the pot and shred them using two forks. Add the chicken shreds back to the saucepan.

4. Add the dried noodles to the pot and cook according to package instructions, usually about 8-10 minutes.

5. Add the chopped bok choy to the pot and cook for an additional 3-4 minutes, or until the bok choy is tender.

6. Add salt and pepper to taste when preparing the soup.

7. Spoon soup into bowls, top with chopped parsley, and serve warm.

Nutritional Value: This soup is low in calories and fat but high in protein and nutrients. The bok choy adds a dose of vitamins A and C, while the chicken provides lean protein.

Cooking Time: Approximately 40 minutes

Servings: 6-8

5. Glorious Strawberry Salad

Ingredients:

- 6 cups mixed salad greens

- 2 cups fresh strawberries, sliced

- 1/2 cup crumbled goat cheese

- 1/4 cup chopped pecans, toasted

- 1/4 cup balsamic vinaigrette

Preparation:

1. In a large bowl, combine the mixed salad greens, sliced strawberries, crumbled goat cheese, and toasted pecans.

2. Drizzle the balsamic vinaigrette over the salad and toss gently to coat all the ingredients.

3. Serve immediately.

Nutritional Value: This salad is packed with antioxidants from the strawberries, healthy fats from the pecans, and protein from the goat cheese. It's also low in calories and a good source of vitamins and minerals.

Preparation Time: 10 minutes

Servings: 4

6. Chicken Tortilla Soup

Ingredients:

- 2 tablespoons olive oil

- 1 onion, diced

- 2 cloves garlic, minced

- 1 jalapeno pepper, seeded and minced

- 1 teaspoon ground cumin

- 1 teaspoon chili powder

- 1 can (14.5 oz) diced tomatoes

- 6 cups chicken broth

- 2 cups cooked shredded chicken.

- 1 canned (15 ounce) black beans, drained and rinsed.

- 1 cup frozen corn kernels

- Salt and pepper to taste

- Tortilla chips, avocado slices, shredded cheese, and chopped cilantro for garnish

Preparation:

1. In a large saucepan, warm the olive oil over medium heat. Add the diced onion, minced garlic, and minced jalapeno pepper. Cook, stirring periodically, until the onion becomes soft and transparent.

2. Stir in the ground cumin and chili powder and cook for an additional minute.

3. Add the diced tomatoes (with their juices), chicken broth, shredded chicken, black beans, and frozen corn kernels to the pot. Bring the soup to a simmer.

4. Allow the soup to boil for 20-25 minutes, stirring periodically.

5. To taste, add pepper and salt to the soup.

6. Ladle the soup into bowls and garnish with tortilla chips, avocado slices, shredded cheese, and chopped cilantro.

Nutritional Value: This soup is a hearty and flavorful meal, rich in protein from the chicken and black beans, and packed with fiber from the vegetables and beans.

Preparation Time: Approximately 45 minutes

Servings: 6-8

7. Shrimp Bisque

Ingredients:

- 1 lb shrimp, peeled and deveined

- 2 tablespoons olive oil

- 1 onion, diced

- 2 carrots, diced

- 2 celery stalks, diced

- 2 cloves garlic, minced

- 1/4 cup tomato paste

- 4 cups fish or shrimp stock

- 1 cup heavy cream

- Salt and pepper to taste

- Fresh parsley for garnish

Preparation:

1. In a large saucepan, warm the olive oil over medium heat. Combine the chopped onion, carrots, celery, and garlic. Cook, stirring periodically, until the veggies have softened.

2. Stir in the tomato paste and cook for an additional 2-3 minutes.

3. Add the shrimp stock to the pot and bring to a simmer.

4. Add the shrimp to the pot and cook for 2-3 minutes, or until they are pink and cooked through.

5. Using a slotted spoon, remove the shrimp from the pot and set aside.

6. Use an immersion blender or transfer the soup to a blender and puree until smooth.

7. Return the soup to the pot, then mix in the heavy cream. Season with salt and pepper to taste.

8. Return the shrimp to the pot and let the soup simmer for an additional 5 minutes.

9. Ladle the soup into bowls, garnish with fresh parsley, and serve hot.

***Nutritional Value:** This creamy bisque is a luxurious treat, rich in protein from the shrimp and dairy, and packed with flavor from the vegetables and herbs.*

Preparation Time: Approximately 45 minutes

Servings: 4-6

CHAPTER 6

Snacks & Desserts

1. Peppered Beef and Citrus Salad

Ingredients:

- One pound of finely sliced beef sirloin.

- Salt and pepper to taste

- 6 cups mixed salad greens

- 2 oranges, peeled and segmented

- 1 grapefruit, peeled and segmented

- 1/4 cup sliced red onion

- 1/4 cup chopped fresh parsley

- 1/4 cup of extra virgin olive oil.

- 2 tablespoons balsamic vinegar

- 1 teaspoon Dijon mustard

Preparation:

1. Season the meat slices with salt and pepper.

2. Heat a skillet over medium-high heat and cook the beef slices for 2-3 minutes on each side until browned and cooked through.

3. In a large bowl, toss together the mixed greens, orange segments, grapefruit segments, red onion, and parsley.

4. In a small bowl, combine the olive oil, balsamic vinegar, and Dijon mustard to create the dressing.

5. Toss the lettuce in the dressing until well coated.

6. Divide the salad onto plates and top with the cooked beef slices.

7. Serve immediately.

Nutritional Value: *This salad is rich in protein from the beef and vitamin C from the citrus fruits. It's also low in carbohydrates and high in healthy fats from the olive oil.*

Cooking Time: Approximately 15 minutes

Number of Servings: 4

2. Orange, Red, and Green Buckwheat Salad

Ingredients:

- 1 cup buckwheat groats

- 2 cups water

- 1 orange, peeled and diced

- 1 red bell pepper, diced

- 1 cup green peas

- 1/4 cup chopped fresh mint

- 1/4 cup crumbled feta cheese

- 2 Tbsp extra virgin olive oil.

- 1 tablespoon lemon juice

- Salt and pepper to taste

Preparation:

1. Rinse the buckwheat groats under cold water and drain.

2. In a saucepan, bring the water to a boil and add the buckwheat groats. Reduce heat to low, cover, and

simmer for 10-12 minutes until the water is absorbed and the buckwheat is tender.

3. In a large bowl, combine the cooked buckwheat, diced orange, diced red bell pepper, green peas, chopped mint, and crumbled feta cheese.

4. In a small bowl, whisk together the olive oil and lemon juice to make the dressing. Season with salt and pepper.

5. Toss the lettuce with the dressing until well coated.

6. Serve the salad cold or at room temperature.

Nutritional Value: *This salad is high in fiber from buckwheat and vegetables, and it provides a good source of vitamin C from the orange and red bell pepper.*

Cooking Time: Approximately 15 minutes

Number of Servings: 4.

3. Baked Papaya and Chicken Salad with Cilantro-Lime Dressing

Ingredients:

- 2 boneless, skinless chicken breasts

- 1 ripe papaya, peeled, seeded, and diced

- 4 cups mixed salad greens

- 1/4 cup chopped red onion

- 1/4 cup chopped fresh cilantro

- 2 tablespoons chopped roasted peanuts

- 2 tablespoons olive oil

- 2 tablespoons lime juice

- 1 teaspoon honey

- Salt and pepper to taste

Preparation:

1. Heat the oven to 375°F (190°C).

2. Season the chicken breasts with salt and pepper and place them on a baking sheet.

3. Bake the chicken breasts for 20-25 minutes until cooked through and no longer pink in the center. Let them cool slightly, then dice into bite-sized pieces.

4. In a large bowl, combine the diced papaya, mixed salad greens, chopped red onion, chopped cilantro, and diced chicken.

5. In a small bowl, whisk together the olive oil, lime juice, honey, salt, and pepper to make the dressing.

6. Pour the dressing over the salad and toss to coat.

7. Sprinkle the chopped roasted peanuts over the salad before serving.

Nutritional Value: *This salad provides lean protein from the chicken, fiber from the papaya and greens, and healthy fats from the olive oil and peanuts. It's also rich in vitamin C and antioxidants from the papaya and cilantro.*

Cooking Time: Approximately 25-30 minutes

4. Chicken Noodle Soup with Bok Choy

Ingredients:

- 6 cups chicken broth

- Thinly slice two boneless and skinless chicken breasts.

- 2 cups sliced bok choy

- 1 cup sliced carrots

- 1 cup sliced celery

- 1 cup cooked noodles (such as egg noodles or rice noodles)

- 2 cloves garlic, minced

- 1 tablespoon grated ginger

- 2 tablespoons soy sauce

- 1 tablespoon sesame oil

- Salt and pepper to taste

- Chopped green onions as garnish (optional).

Preparation:

1. In a large saucepan, bring the chicken broth to a simmer over medium heat.

2. Add the sliced chicken breasts, bok choy, carrots, celery, garlic, and ginger to the pot. Simmer for 10-15 minutes until the chicken is cooked through and the vegetables are tender.

3. Stir in the cooked noodles, soy sauce, and sesame oil. Season with salt and pepper to taste.

4. Ladle the soup into bowls and garnish with chopped green onions if desired.

Nutritional Value: This soup is low in fat and calories but high in protein from the chicken and contains a good amount of vitamins and minerals from the vegetables.

Cooking Time: Approximately 25-30 minutes

Number of Servings: 4-6

5. Glorious Strawberry Salad

Ingredients:

- 6 cups mixed salad greens

- 2 cups sliced strawberries

- 1/2 cup crumbled feta cheese

- 1/4 cup sliced almonds

- 1/4 cup balsamic vinegar

- 2 Tbsps. extra virgin olive oil.

- 1 tablespoon honey

- Salt and pepper to taste

Preparation:

1. In a large bowl, combine the mixed salad greens, sliced strawberries, crumbled feta cheese, and sliced almonds.

2. In a small bowl, whisk together the balsamic vinegar, olive oil, honey, salt, and pepper to make the dressing.

3. Toss the salad in the dressing until well coated.

4. Serve immediately.

Nutritional Value: *This salad is packed with vitamins, minerals, and antioxidants from the mixed greens and strawberries. It also provides healthy fats from the olive oil and protein from the feta cheese and almonds.*

Preparation Time: Approximately 10 minutes
Number of Servings: 4

6. Chicken Tortilla Soup:

Ingredients:

- 1 tablespoon olive oil

- 1 onion, diced

- 2 cloves garlic, minced

- 1 jalapeño, seeded and diced

- 1 teaspoon ground cumin

- 1 teaspoon chili powder

- 4 cups chicken broth

- 1 can (14.5 oz) diced tomatoes

- 1 cup corn kernels, fresh or frozen.

- 1 cup black beans, drained and rinsed

- 2 cups cooked shredded chicken

- Salt and pepper to taste

- Tortilla chips, sliced avocado, shredded cheese, and chopped cilantro for garnish (optional)

Preparation:

1. In a large saucepan, warm the olive oil over medium heat. Add diced onion, garlic, and jalapeño. Cook for 5 minutes until softened.

2. Stir in the ground cumin and chili powder and cook for another minute until fragrant.

3. Add the chicken broth and diced tomatoes with their juices. Bring the soup to a simmer.

4. Add the corn kernels, black beans, and shredded chicken to the pot. Heat for 15-20 minutes to let the flavors combine.

5. Season the soup with salt and pepper as desired.

6. Ladle the soup into bowls and garnish with tortilla chips, sliced avocado, shredded cheese, and chopped cilantro if desired.

Nutritional Value: This soup is rich in protein from the chicken and black beans, and it provides fiber and vitamins from the vegetables. It's low in fat and can be customized with various toppings for added flavor.

Cooking Time: Approximately 30 minutes
Number of Servings: 4-6

7. Shrimp Bisque

Ingredients:

- 1 pound of shrimp, peeled and deveined.

- Four cups of seafood or chicken broth.

- 1 onion, diced

- 2 carrots, diced

- 2 celery stalks, diced

- 2 cloves garlic, minced

- 1/4 cup tomato paste

- 1/2 cup heavy cream

- 2 tablespoons butter

- 2 tablespoons all-purpose flour

- Salt and pepper to taste

- Chopped fresh parsley for garnish

Preparation:

1. In a large saucepan, melt the butter over medium heat. Add the diced onion, carrots, celery, and garlic. Cook for 5-7 minutes until softened.

2. Stir in the tomato paste and simmer for a further 2 minutes.

3. Sprinkle the flour over the vegetables and cook for 1-2 minutes to create a roux.

4. Gradually whisk in the seafood or chicken broth, stirring constantly to prevent lumps from forming.

5. Bring the soup to a simmer and add the shrimp. Cook for 3-4 minutes, or until the shrimp become pink and are fully cooked.

6. Stir in the heavy cream, then season with salt and pepper to taste.

7. Ladle the bisque into bowls and garnish with chopped fresh parsley before serving.

Nutritional Value: *This bisque is creamy and indulgent, with the richness of shrimp and cream balanced by the vegetables. It's high in protein and provides essential vitamins and minerals.*

Cooking Time: Approximately 30 minutes

Number of Servings: 4-6

CONCLUSION

In conclusion, "The Complete Low-FODMAP Diet Cookbook for Beginners 2024" offers a comprehensive guide to navigating the low-FODMAP diet, providing a wide range of delicious and nutritious recipes suitable for individuals with digestive sensitivities. By understanding and implementing the principles of the low-FODMAP diet, you can effectively manage symptoms such as bloating, gas, and abdominal pain, thereby improving your overall quality of life.

This cookbook presents a diverse selection of recipes, from flavorful salads and soups to hearty main dishes and satisfying snacks, ensuring that individuals following the low-FODMAP diet never feel deprived or restricted in their culinary options. Each recipe is carefully crafted to be low in fermentable carbohydrates, making them gentle on the digestive system while still being packed with essential nutrients and vibrant flavors.

Moreover, this cookbook serves as an invaluable resource for beginners embarking on their low-FODMAP journey, offering detailed explanations of FODMAPs, guidance on how to identify trigger foods and practical tips for grocery shopping and meal planning. With clear instructions and helpful nutritional information accompanying each recipe, readers can feel confident in their ability to successfully implement the low-FODMAP diet into their daily lives.

As individuals embrace the low-FODMAP diet and experience relief from their digestive symptoms, they are empowered to take control of their health and well-being. By nourishing their bodies with wholesome, gut-friendly foods, readers can cultivate a greater sense of vitality and vitality, allowing them to fully engage in all aspects of life with renewed energy and vitality.

In adopting and adapting to the low-FODMAP diet, readers not only improve their health but also inspire others to prioritize digestive wellness. By making conscious choices to support their digestive systems, individuals set a powerful example of self-care and resilience, demonstrating the transformative impact that dietary interventions can have on overall health and vitality. Embracing the low-FODMAP diet is not just about managing symptoms; it's about reclaiming control over one's health and embracing a lifestyle of vitality and well-being.

BONUS

14 Days Meal Plan

Day 1:

- Breakfast: Omelette with spinach, tomatoes, and cheddar cheese

- Snack: Carrot sticks with lactose-free yogurt dip

- Lunch: Grilled chicken salad with mixed greens, cucumber, and a lemon vinaigrette

- Snack: Rice cakes with peanut butter (ensure it's made with just peanuts).

- Dinner: baked salmon, quinoa, and boiled green beans.

Day 2:

- Breakfast: Smoothie made with lactose-free yogurt, banana (ensure it's ripe), and strawberries

- Snack: Hard-boiled eggs

- Lunch: Turkey wrap with lettuce, tomato, and lactose-free cheese in a gluten-free tortilla

- Snack: Mixed nuts (almonds, walnuts, and pecans)

- Dinner: Stir-fried tofu with bell peppers, zucchini, and rice noodles

Day 3:

- Breakfast: Gluten-free oats with almond milk, topped with strawberries and a sprinkle of chia seeds

- Snack: Sliced cucumber with hummus (ensure it's made without garlic or onion)

- Lunch: Quinoa salad with grilled shrimp, arugula, cherry tomatoes, and a balsamic vinaigrette

- Snack: Rice crackers with tuna salad (made with canned tuna, mayo, and mustard)

- Dinner: Grilled steak with roasted potatoes and sautéed spinach

Day 4:

- Breakfast: Scrambled eggs with spinach, bell peppers, and lactose-free cheese

- Snack: Popcorn (plain, without added flavorings)

- Lunch: Chicken and vegetable soup with homemade chicken broth

- Snack: Strawberries with lactose-free whipped cream

- Dinner: Baked cod with quinoa pilaf and steamed carrots

Day 5:

- Breakfast: Greek yogurt parfait with lactose-free yogurt, blueberries, and granola (ensure it's low FODMAP)

- Snack: Rice cakes with almond butter

- Lunch: Turkey and avocado lettuce wraps with sliced tomato and cucumber

- Snack: Mixed berries (strawberries, raspberries, and blueberries)

- Dinner: Grilled chicken breast with mashed potatoes and steamed green beans.

Day 6:

- Breakfast: Smoothie made with lactose-free yogurt, kiwi (peeled), and pineapple

- Snack: Rice crackers with lactose-free cream cheese

- Lunch: Quinoa salad with grilled tofu, baby spinach, cherry tomatoes, and a lemon tahini dressing

- Snack: Sliced bell peppers with guacamole

- Dinner: Baked pork chops with roasted sweet potatoes and steamed broccoli.

Day 7:

- Breakfast: Scrambled eggs with tomatoes, spinach, and lactose-free cheese

- Snack: Mixed nuts (cashews, almonds, and walnuts)

- Lunch: Grilled salmon with a side of quinoa salad (quinoa, cucumber, red bell pepper, and parsley)

- Snack: Rice cakes with peanut butter

- Dinner: Stir-fried beef with bok choy, carrots, and rice noodles.

Day 8:

- Breakfast: Gluten-free toast with scrambled eggs and sautéed spinach

- Snack: Carrot sticks with lactose-free yogurt dip

- Lunch: Turkey and cranberry sandwich with gluten-free bread and mixed greens

- Snack: Rice cakes with almond butter

- Dinner: Grilled chicken skewers with bell peppers and pineapple, served with jasmine rice

Day 9:

- Breakfast: Smoothie made with lactose-free yogurt, strawberries, and banana (ensure it's ripe)

- Snack: Hard-boiled eggs

- Lunch: Tuna salad with mixed leaves, cherry tomatoes, and balsamic vinaigrette.

- Snack: Rice crackers with lactose-free cream cheese

- Dinner: Baked cod with roasted potatoes and steamed green beans

Day 10:

- Breakfast: Greek yogurt parfait with lactose-free yogurt, blueberries, and gluten-free granola

- Snack: Mixed nuts (almonds, pecans, and walnuts)

- Lunch: Quinoa salad with grilled shrimp, arugula, cherry tomatoes, and a lemon vinaigrette

- Snack: Sliced cucumber with hummus

- Dinner: Grilled steak with mashed potatoes and sautéed spinach.

Day 11:

- Breakfast: Omelette with spinach, tomatoes, and lactose-free cheese

- Snack: Rice cakes with peanut butter

- Lunch: Turkey and avocado wrap with lettuce, tomato, and lactose-free cheese in a gluten-free tortilla

- Snack: Mixed berries (strawberries, raspberries, and blueberries)

- Dinner: Baked salmon with quinoa pilaf and steamed carrots.

Day 12:

- Breakfast: Smoothie made with lactose-free yogurt, kiwi (peeled), and pineapple

- Snack: Carrot sticks with lactose-free yogurt dip

- Lunch: Grilled chicken salad with mixed greens, cucumber, and a lemon vinaigrette

- Snack: Hard-boiled eggs

- Dinner: Stir-fried tofu with bell peppers, zucchini, and rice noodles

Day 13:

- Breakfast: Gluten-free oats with almond milk, topped with strawberries and a sprinkle of chia seeds

- Snack: Rice crackers with lactose-free cream cheese

- Lunch: Chicken and vegetable soup with homemade chicken broth

- Snack: Popcorn (plain, without added flavorings)

- Dinner: Grilled steak with roasted potatoes and sautéed spinach

Day 14:

- Breakfast: Scrambled eggs with tomatoes, spinach, and lactose-free cheese

- Snack: Sliced bell peppers with hummus

- Lunch: Quinoa salad with grilled tofu, baby spinach, cherry tomatoes, and a lemon tahini dressing

- Snack: Mixed nuts (cashews, almonds, and walnuts)

- Dinner: Baked pork chops with mashed potatoes and steamed green beans.